THE NEW ULTIMATE

VOLUMETRICS DIET PLAN

105 Delicious Low Calories Recipes for Sustainable Weight Loss

PATRICK BRYANT

Table of Contents

INTRODUCTION

The Volumetrics diet was developed by Dr. Barbara Rolls, a nutrition professor at Penn State University, with the intention of creating a dietary approach that emphasizes healthy eating patterns rather than a structured, restrictive diet.

The Volumetrics series of books is centered around dietary "energy density" and "nutrient density." Foods with high energy density have a higher calorie content in a given portion, while those with low energy density have fewer calories per portion. Similarly, foods that are nutrient-dense provide high levels of nutrients relative to the calories they contain, often having little or no saturated fat, sodium or added sugars.

The Volumetrics diet emphasizes eating low-energy-dense, high-nutrient-dense foods like fruits, vegetables, whole grains and low-fat dairy. Conversely, high-energy-dense foods, such as those with a high proportion of unhealthy fats or sugar and little moisture, are recommended to be limited. The idea is that by focusing on eating foods that are lower in calories and higher in water and important nutrients like fiber, the body will feel satisfied while still losing weight.

Guidelines for the Volumetrics diet

Instead of singling out specific foods or food groups to avoid, the Volumetrics philosophy is more about what to eat. Foods are divided into four groups based on their energy density that help with meal planning and portion control.

Group 1: Foods including non-starchy fruits and vegetables, nonfat milk and broth-based soups

Group 2: Foods including starchy fruits and vegetables, grains, breakfast cereal, low-fat meat, legumes and low-fat mixed dishes

Group 3: Foods including meat, cheese, pizza, French fries, salad dressing, bread, pretzels, ice cream and cake

Group 4: Foods including crackers, chips, chocolate candies, cookies, nuts, butter and oil.

Foods contained within Group 1 are very low in energy density and are considered "free" foods to eat any time.

The energy density increases from Groups 2 to 4, so more attention to portion control is needed with foods in these groups to avoid excess energy intake. Portion sizes and specific inclusion of groups will vary from person to person, but most will fall into a similar pattern of three meals and two to three snacks each day. Followers of the Volumetrics diet can keep track of what they eat and drink in a food record to monitor progress and identify common patterns, but exact measurements aren't required. In addition to the food component, the Volumetrics diet provides specific plans for increasing exercise to at least 30 minutes per day most days of the week, an amount supported by the 2018 Physical Activity Guidelines for Americans.

One of the benefits of the Volumetrics diet is that it doesn't put any foods on a "do not eat" list, which gives people the freedom to choose where high-nutrient-dense foods and drinks fit within their overall eating pattern. Some research suggests that the more we restrict a particular food or food group, the more we want it, so building in "room" for certain favorites offers a healthier way of framing caloric splurges. Specifically, small portions of foods considered to be healthy and energy-dense, like common cooking oils (e.g., olive and canola oils) and nuts (e.g., almonds and walnuts), are recommended. These foods provide essential fatty acids that our bodies use for vitamin and mineral absorption, energy production and maintaining cell health; and this diet acknowledges that they are important to include rather than skip altogether.

What Is the Volumetrics Diet?

The volumetrics diet emphasizes eating nutrient-dense, low-calorie foods, such as fruits, vegetables, whole grains and low-fat dairy. Lower calorie foods have high water content, which adds volume to food and helps people feel sated. These are mostly water-rich foods, like fruits and non-starchy vegetables or broth-based soups. The diet encourages limiting high-calorie density foods, including foods with a high proportion of unhealthy fats and added sugar. The eating regimen, pioneered by Penn State University nutrition professor Barbara Rolls, is more of an approach to eating than it is a structured diet.

With "The Volumetrics Diet" book as your guide, you'll learn to recognize a food's caloric density, cut the calorie density of your meals and make choices that fight hunger. "The book emphasizes thinking positively about what you can eat," Rolls says. "It doesn't say don't eat higher-calorie density foods. It says you should manage portions to meet your calorie goals. If you choose lower-calorie density foods you get a bigger portion for whatever calorie amount you are intending to eat or should be eating."

• Family friendly. Family members can easily eat all the meals together with little or no modification. The food options are healthy and balanced enough for all ages.

• Budget friendly. Foods for this diet are easy to find at a typical grocery and don't require expensive or specialty food items.

• Planet friendly. This diet considers the environmental effects of food choices. It's largely plant-based and/or the foods are mainly sustainably grown/produced.

• Vegan or vegetarian friendly. Recipes can be easily modified for a vegan or vegetarian diet.

• Gluten-free friendly. Recipes can be easily modified and still follow a gluten-free diet.

• Halal friendly. Recipes can be easily modified and still follow the diet.

• Kosher friendly. Recipes can be easily modified and still follow the diet.

• Low-carb. This diet recommends limiting sugary beverages and other foods high in refined carbohydrates.

• Low-fat. This diet emphasizes foods that have little to no saturated fat.

The Volumetrics diet and health

While more analysis is needed on the role of energy density in weight management and the prevention of overweight and obesity, there is research supporting the use of a low-energy-dense diet to improve appetite control and help achieve weight-loss goals. By emphasizing whole foods and personalization of the diet rather than cutting out entire food groups or placing strict rules on food consumption, the Volumetrics diet is likely to be a more sustainable eating pattern than popular, quick-fix fad diets.

Some research has also been done on the connection between energy density and specific health outcomes:

• Cardiovascular disease: Some research suggeststhe potential for a low-energy-dense diet to benefit factors affecting cardiovascular disease, but sufficient evidence is lacking to fully support this.

• Type 2 diabetes: In a large observational study, women who ate diets higher in energy density had a higher risk of developing type 2 diabetes as compared with women who followed a lower-energy-dense diet.

• Breast cancer: One large observational study determined that women who had the highest-energy-dense diet had a higher risk for postmenopausal breast cancer compared with women who followed the lowest energy-dense diet.

• Weight loss: Several systematic reviews and meta-analyses of observational studies have found lower-energy-dense diets to be associated with lower body weights. Evidence from randomized controlled trials have also shown lower-energy-dense diets to be helpful for weight management and weight loss maintenance.

Most of these condition-specific studies have been observational in design, meaning that they can't prove cause and effect like randomized controlled trials (RCTs) can (that is, that a lower-energy-dense diet caused a lower risk for disease development). Studies on the impact of energy density on body weight have been tested in RCTs with positive results. That said, larger and longer-term RCTs are needed to fully understand the effects of energy density on specific health conditions and in different populations.

The Science Behind the Volumetric Approach

Volumetric analysis is a chemical analytical procedure based on measurement of volumes of reaction in solutions. It uses titration to determine the concentration of a solution by carefully measuring the volume of one solution needed to react with another. In this process, a measured volume of a standard solution, the titrant, is added from a burette to the solution of unknown concentration. When the two substances are present in exact stoichiometric ratio, the reaction is said to have reached the equivalence or stoichiometric point.

In order to determine when this occurs, another substance, the indicator, is also added to the reaction mixture. This is an organic dye which changes color when the reaction is complete. This color change is known as the end point; ideally, it will coincide with the equivalence point. For various reasons, there is usually some difference between the two, though if the indicator is carefully chosen, the difference will be negligible. A typical titration is based on a reaction of the general type $aA + bB \rightarrow$ products where A is the titrant, B the substance titrated, and a:b is the stoichiometric ratio between the two. Some indicators include Litmus, Methyl Orange, Methyl Red, Phenolphthalein, and Thymol Blue. Titration can be applied to any of the following chemical reactions: • Acid–base • Complexation • Oxidation–reduction • Precipitation Only acid–base and oxidation–reduction titration will be treated here, though the fundamental principles are the same in all cases. Acid–base titration involves measuring the volume of a solution of the acid (or base) that is required to completely react with a known volume of a solution of a base (or acid). The relative amounts of acid and base required to reach the equivalence point depend on their stoichiometric coefficients. It is therefore critical to have a balanced equation before attempting calculations based on acid–base reactions. Below we define some of the common terms associated with acid–base reactions.

A molar solution is one that contains one mole of the substance per liter of solution. For example, a molar solution of sodium hydroxide contains 40 g ($NaOH=40$ g/mol) of the solute per liter of solution. As described in chapter 13, the concentration of a solution expressed in moles per liter of solution is known as the molarity of the solution.

Foods to eat and avoid

Rather than banning any foods entirely, the Volumetrics Diet divides them into four categories based on their calorie density.

Category 1

Foods in Category 1 have a very low calorie density and should comprise the majority of your diet. They include:
• Fruits: apples, oranges, pears, peaches, bananas, berries, and grapefruit
• Non-starchy vegetables: broccoli, cauliflower, carrots, tomatoes, zucchini, and kale
• Soups: broth-based soups like vegetable soup, chicken soup, minestrone, and lentil soup
• Nonfat dairy: skim milk and nonfat yogurt
• Beverages: water, black coffee, and unsweetened tea

Category 2
Foods in the second category have a low energy density and can be enjoyed in moderation. They include:
• Whole grains: quinoa, couscous, farro, buckwheat, barley, and brown rice
• Legumes: chickpeas, lentils, black beans, and kidney beans
• Starchy vegetables: potatoes, corn, peas, squash, and parsnips
• Lean proteins: skinless poultry, white fish, and lean cuts of beef or pork

Category 3
Foods in the third category are considered medium calorie density. While they're permitted, it's important to keep an eye on serving sizes. These foods include:
• Meat: fatty fish, poultry with the skin, and high fat cuts of pork and beef
• Refined carbs: white bread, white rice, crackers, and white pasta
• Full fat dairy: whole milk, full fat yogurt, ice cream, and cheese

Category 4

Foods in the final category are classified as high energy density. These foods contain lots of calories per serving and should be eaten sparingly. They include:
• Nuts: almonds, walnuts, macadamia nuts, pecans, and pistachios
• Seeds: chia seeds, sesame seeds, hemp seeds, and flax seeds
• Oils: butter, vegetable oil, olive oil, margarine, and lard
• Processed foods: cookies, candies, chips, pretzels, and fast food

Sample 3-day meal plan

On the Volumetrics Diet, you should eat 3 meals per day, plus 2–3 snacks. Here's a 3-day sample menu:
Day 1
• Breakfast: oatmeal with fruit and a glass of skim milk
• Snack: carrots with hummus
• Lunch: grilled chicken with quinoa and asparagus
• Snack: sliced apples and light string cheese
• Dinner: baked cod with spiced vegetable couscous
Day 2
• Breakfast: nonfat yogurt with strawberries and blueberries
• Snack: a hard-boiled egg with tomato slices
• Lunch: turkey chili with kidney beans and vegetables
• Snack: a fruit salad with melon, kiwi, and strawberries
• Dinner: zucchini boats stuffed with ground beef, tomatoes, bell peppers, and marinara sauce
Day 3

• Breakfast: scrambled eggs with mushrooms, tomatoes, and onions, plus a slice of whole wheat toast
• Snack: a smoothie with skim milk, banana, and berries
• Lunch: chicken noodle soup with a side salad
• Snack: air-popped popcorn
• Dinner: whole grain pasta with turkey meatballs and sautéed vegetables

How Does the Volumetrics Diet Plan Work?

Volumetrics places the emphasis on eating rather than deprivation. "The focus is 100 percent about fullness," says Chicago-based Dawn Jackson Blatner, RD, author of The Flexitarian Diet and The Superfood Swap. "This diet is trying to get you full because, when given a choice, people will choose to eat more."

According to Volumetrics, foods that contain more water, such as fruits and vegetables, are healthier because they have lower energy density, or number of calories in a specific amount of food, than other options that have comparable satiety. Foods that have high energy density include sugary and fatty foods, such as potato chips and cookies. "[Rolls] is saying that you can naturally turn off your desire for these foods," says Blatner.

Essentially, the claim that advocates of Volumetrics make is you can lose weight by eating fewer calories yet still feel full. Volumetrics is one of my favorite diets because it's more about eating than dieting," says Andrea Giancoli, MPH, RD, a nutrition communications consultant based in

Hermosa Beach, California. "People like to eat, and research has shown that when you eat high-water-content foods, such as a green salad with a lot of vegetables or soup, you eat less [calories]." Volumetrics also gives tools to calculate the energy density of foods, and recommends using a food journal and getting enough physical activity. "Research shows that keeping a food journal is one of the tactics that work for successful weight loss," says Giancoli.

Is Volumetrics Easy to Follow?

Volumetrics isn't restrictive and should be relatively easy to follow. Most – if not all – of the foods you'd eat on the diet are available at most grocery stores.
You won't go hungry on volumetrics. Daily menus are designed to be filling and include snacks and dessert. The focus is on making smart, sustainable tweaks to your eating habits that lower the overall caloric density of your diet. Since volumetrics doesn't ban or restrict entire food groups, your chances of sticking with it are higher. Volumetrics offers convenience. You're free to eat out as long as you follow the diet's guidelines, but cooking is encouraged for best results. Alcohol is allowed in moderation. Volumetrics books offer guidance and ideas to make the plan easier.
There are plenty of volumetrics recipes to choose from. Hundreds of recipes for appetizers, soups, sandwiches, pasta and vegetarian dishes (modified to cut caloric density) are included in Rolls' books.
Eating out is allowed by the volumetrics approach. You'll have to determine which menu choices are the best to stick with your volumetrics diet. Starting with a low-calorie soup

or salad will help make you less likely to order a large entrée.

Feeling full shouldn't be an issue. Volumetrics was designed to help you feel full and satiated. You shouldn't feel hungry on the diet, provided you adhere to its guidelines. Fruits, vegetables, soup and other low-density foods help control appetite, as do lean protein choices like poultry, seafood, tofu and beans.

There's no need to compromise on taste. You don't have to give up your favorites with volumetrics – just make smart changes. If you leave the butter off your bread, for example, you can have two slices instead of one for the same amount of calories. Choose skim milk instead of whole milk. And a morning stack of pancakes is still OK, as long as you switch to whole-wheat flour, cut the oil and butter and add fresh fruit on top instead of adding syrup. Other meal ideas range from a baked potato topped with vegetables, salsa and cheese to chicken fajita pizza.

What the Science Says About Whether Volumetrics Works

A number of studies have examined how energy density of food — or the ratio between how much energy (calories) a food provides and how much it weighs — can affect weight loss and weight maintenance. For example, a carrot, which contains a lot of water, would have a low energy density, since it does not contain a lot of calories for how much it weighs.

One study found that eating a diet with a lower energy density, including more vegetables and whole grains, could help people maintain their weight loss. A 2016 review looked at 13 studies and found evidence that suggested that paying attention to the energy density of food could help people with obesity manage their weight.

A Sample Food List for the Volumetrics Diet

The Volumetrics diet plan is not about telling you what you can and can't eat, but rather aims to teach you how to eat and stay satisfied. That said, the program does recommend certain foods that have high water content (low energy density), high fiber, and high nutrient density, to help promote satiety. These foods include:
• Fresh fruits (rather than dried fruit or juice, for example)
• Fresh or frozen vegetables (try swapping some in for half a portion of pasta in a pasta dish, for example)
• Beans and legumes
• Whole grains
• Fiber-rich breakfast cereals
• Low-fat fish
• Poultry without skin
• Lean meats
• Minimal added sugars
• Water (rather than sugary drinks)

A 1-Day Sample Menu of the Volumetrics Diet Plan
This sample meal shows that there is a high volume of good food on this diet:
Breakfast

• Oatmeal topped with apple slices, cinnamon, and a sprinkle of brown sugar
• Nonfat milk
• ½ grapefruit
• Coffee
Lunch
• Grilled chicken salad with chopped romaine lettuce, red bell pepper, 1 teaspoon crumbled blue cheese, and chopped walnuts with light dressing
• Whole-wheat pita bread
• Strawberries
Snack
• Cheerios with skim milk and fresh blueberries
Dinner
• Steak fajita with grilled green peppers and onions, salsa, shredded romaine lettuce, diced fresh tomato, corn kernels, and nonfat sour cream on a tortilla
• Cantaloupe

The Potential Health Benefits of the Volumetrics Diet Plan

So should you consider trying the Volumetrics diet to help curb your appetite and improve your health? Certainly, Volumetrics has some distinct advantages:

• Solid Science "Volumetrics is sound advice that is backed by research," says Giancoli. "The diet comes with science behind it."

• Good Foods A big advantage of Volumetrics is the emphasis on learning how to eat water-rich foods, such as fruits and vegetables, which tend to be healthier foods. "It's one of the best concepts out there because it teaches you how to eat right," says Blatner. "It promotes all the healthy foods we know."

• No Crash Dieting Rolls' books on Volumetrics promote a safe and slow loss of 1 to 2 lbs a week, aiming for sustainable rather than rapid weight loss.

• No Rigid Rules When you start this diet, you won't have to tell yourself that you're never having chocolate or cheese again — instead, you'll learn how to work it into your diet in the most healthful way possible.

How volumetric diet works

The Volumetrics Diet groups foods into four categories based on their calorie density:

• Category 1 (very low calorie density): calorie density of less than 0.6

• Category 2 (low calorie density): calorie density of 0.6–1.5

• Category 3 (medium calorie density): calorie density of 1.6–3.9

• Category 4 (high calorie density): calorie density of 4.0–9.0

Dr. Rolls's book provides detailed information on how to calculate calorie density. In general, you should divide the number of calories in a particular serving size by its weight in grams. You'll end up with a figure between 0 and 9. Foods with a high water content, such as broccoli, typically score very low in calorie density, while desserts and processed foods like dark chocolate usually rank high. A typical meal on the Volumetrics Diet should mostly comprise foods from Category 1, as well as include foods from Category 2 to help round out your plate. You can eat small amounts of foods from Category 3 and very limited portions from Category 4.

The diet's standard meal plan provides around 1,400 calories per day but can be adjusted to fit your calorie goals by adding extra snacks or increasing portion sizes. No foods are completely off-limits on the Volumetrics Diet. In fact, you can include foods with a high calorie density by modifying your portion sizes and adjusting your other meals.

Furthermore, the diet encourages at least 30–60 minutes of exercise each day.

You should keep track of your physical activity and food intake in a journal to monitor your progress and identify areas that may need improvement.

Does it work for weight loss?

Although few studies have examined the Volumetrics Diet specifically, research suggests that its central tenets aid weight loss.

Promotes low calorie intake

Selecting foods with a low calorie density is particularly effective. Because these foods have a substantial volume but are low in calories, you can eat large servings without significantly increasing your calorie intake. Notably, a review of 13 studies in 3,628 people tied foods with a lower calorie density to increased weight loss. Similarly, an 8-year study in over 50,000 women associated high-calorie-density foods with increased weight gain. Choosing foods with a low calorie density may also help curb cravings and reduce appetite, which could boost weight loss. A 12-week study in 96 women with excess weight and obesity found that meals with a lower calorie density led to decreased cravings, increased feelings of fullness, and reduced hunger.

In an older study in 39 women, participants ate 56% more calories when served a large portion of a high-calorie-density meal, compared with a smaller, low-calorie-density meal

Encourages regular exercise

Exercise is another important component of the Volumetrics Diet.
The diet recommends getting at least 30–60 minutes of physical activity per day, which may increase weight loss and fat loss by raising your energy expenditure, or the number of calories burned during the day

Other health benefits

The Volumetrics Diet may offer several other health benefits.

May boost diet quality

By encouraging healthy foods that are low in calories but high in fiber, vitamins, and minerals, the Volumetrics Diet may help increase your intake of key nutrients and protect against nutritional deficiencies.

What's more, some research links diets with a low calorie density to improved diet quality.

Limits processed foods

Although the Volumetrics Diet doesn't completely ban any foods, most processed foods have a high calorie density and should be restricted as part of the plan.
Processed foods are not only typically lacking in essential nutrients like fiber, protein, vitamins, and minerals but also usually higher in calories, fat, sugar, and sodium.
Furthermore, studies tie regular intake of processed foods to a higher risk of cancer, heart disease, and premature death.

Flexible and sustainable

Unlike most fad diets, the Volumetrics Diet should be viewed as a long-term lifestyle change.
It pushes you to become more aware of your eating habits and food choices, which can help you make healthier dietary decisions by prioritizing foods with a lower calorie density, such as fruits and vegetables.
Additionally, because no foods are banned on the diet, you can enjoy your favorite dishes by making modifications and adjustments to your diet.
This may make the Volumetrics Diet a good fit for people seeking some flexibility and a sustainable eating plan to follow long term.

Potential downsides of Volumetrics diet

The Volumetrics Diet has a few drawbacks to be aware of.
Time-intensive with few online resources
The diet requires significant time and energy investments, which may make it untenable for some people. In addition to finding recipes, planning meals, and calculating calorie density, you're supposed to prepare most of your meals and snacks at home. This may make the diet too restrictive for those with a busy lifestyle, cramped kitchen, or limited access to fresh produce. Although some support groups and recipes are available, online apps and resources for the diet are somewhat limited. In fact, you may need to purchase the book by Dr. Rolls to calculate your meals' calorie density and track your food intake effectively.

Limits healthy fats

The diet also restricts certain foods rich in healthy fats, including nuts, seeds, and oils.
These foods provide monounsaturated and polyunsaturated fats, which may reduce inflammation and safeguard against chronic conditions like heart disease. Moreover, many nutritious eating patterns like the Mediterranean diet encourage you to eat these foods.

Places too much emphasis on calories

Given that the Volumetrics Diet is based on calorie density, high calorie foods are limited.
This means that nutritious, high calorie foods like avocados, nut butter, and whole eggs are limited, while

processed, low calorie foods like fat-free salad dressing and diet ice cream are allowed due to their low calorie density. Low calorie foods are often packed with added sugar and other unhealthy ingredients to enhance their taste. Just because something is low in calories doesn't mean it's healthy.

The four categories of Volumetrics diet

The Volumetrics diet breaks food down into four categories. To determine which category a food belongs in, you divide the number of calories per serving by its weight in grams. The result is a number between zero and nine.

If you're attempting to lose weight on the Volumetrics diet, you're encouraged to eat 1,400 calories a day. The majority of what you eat in a day should be coming from categories one and two, but occasional, small indulges from categories three and four are acceptable.

1. Category one (calorie density under 0.6): This category of food forms the foundation of your diet. In other words, this is the stuff you fill up on. These foods — due to their high water content — should help you feel full. A few examples of category one foods are:

• Fruits like bananas, apples and grapefruit.

• Non-starchy vegetables like broccoli, carrots, beets and Brussels sprouts.

• Nonfat dairy products like nonfat yogurt or skim milk. (If you aren't a dairy drinker, never fear: Most unsweetened milk substitutes also fall into this category.)

• Broth-based soups of all sorts.

2. Category two (calorie density 0.7 to 1.5): This category contains foods that are healthy when consumed in moderation. A few examples of category two foods are:
• Skinless chicken and turkey and lean cuts of pork or beef.
• Legumes: lentils, chickpeas and dried beans.
• Starchy vegetables: corn, potatoes and squash.
• Whole grains: brown rice, quinoa and farro.
3. Category three (calorie density 1.6 to 3.9): This category contains food that, while still fairly healthy, should only be consumed in small portions. A few examples of category three foods are:
• Fatty meat and fish, as well as skin-on poultry.
• Full-fat dairy products such as ice cream, cheese and whole milk.
• Refined carbohydrates like pasta, white bread and white rice.
4. Category four (calorie density 4 to 9): This category includes processed, sugary and fatty foods, which should be eaten very sparingly. A few examples of category four foods are:
• Nuts and seeds.
• Oils, butter and shortening.
• Fast food, candy and chips.

Pros and cons of the Volumetrics diet

When it comes to weight loss and nutrition, one size doesn't fit all. Zumpano explains that choosing the diet that's right for you is a personal process.

"It's affected by the foods you enjoy, and know that you can't give up, food availability, and how motivated you are to make changes to your eating habits and food choices," she says.

Here are some commonly stated benefits and drawbacks of the Volumetrics diet:

Pros
• Promotes long-term healthy eating. The Volumetrics diet is designed to be sustainable and healthy in the long term. It's sort of a "come for the weight loss, stay for the health benefits" kind of situation.
• Weight loss is long-term. Short-term diets often cause your weight to yo-yo back and forth. Because the Volumetrics diet is intended to be a permanent lifestyle change, those who follow the plan may lose weight a bit slower, but have a good shot at keeping it off.
• No foods are "off-limits." Go ahead and have a small slice of birthday cake. If you're craving pretzels, have some. While you have to limit the quantity of category four foods you're eating, nothing is prohibited.
• Accessible to everybody. Are you vegan? Do you keep kosher? Have you been diagnosed with celiac disease? That's OK Because there aren't any hard and fast restrictions in the Volumetrics diet, you can eat — or not eat — according to your needs.
• It's safe! Volumetrics isn't a fad diet. It doesn't ask you to maintain a dangerously high-calorie deficit, eliminate entire categories of food from your diet or cultivate a negative relationship with food. You don't have to cook separate meals for yourself and your children because you aren't consuming "diet food." You're just living a healthy lifestyle.
• There are lots of resources at your disposal. Besides the four books the diet's creator already penned, there's a lot of

scientific research supporting the plan, and plenty of websites devoted to recipes.

Cons
While most doctors and dietitians agree that it's a solid approach, the Volumetrics diet isn't perfect. Here are some of the downsides to the program:
• It limits the consumption of healthy fats. Millennials beware: Volumetrics is coming for your avocado toast! The Volumetrics diet doesn't distinguish between healthy and unhealthy fats like some other eating plans do. As a result, nuts and seeds occupy the same category (four) as candy and fast food.
• It may be too calorie-focused. Energy-density calculation is the basis of the Volumetrics diet, which means calorie counting is foundational to the plan. Over time, we've learned that calorie counting isn't foolproof. It can often treat foods that have the same amount of calories — such as 1 ounce of nuts and 1 ounce of chips — as nutritional equivalents. We now know all calories aren't created equally. As Zumpano puts it, "Even if weight loss is your goal, caloric restriction is not the only way to get towards weight loss." The good news is, there are ways to deemphasize caloric intake. More on that later.
• It's a big-time commitment. The Volumetrics diet isn't microwave-meal friendly. The emphasis on fresh fruit and vegetables over processed foods makes the diet a healthy choice. But it also makes the plan hard to follow without regular trips to the grocery store and a lot of home cooking. If you decide to go full-bore on the food journaling and energy-density calculation, that will also take some time.
• It can get boring. All that soup is eventually going to get a little dull. If your meals are starting to feel a bit predictable

you can spice things up — literally — by adding new recipes into your rotation.

• Eating out is difficult. While many chain restaurants can make nutrition information available to you on request, the chef isn't likely to hand over the recipe. Without that information, categorizing and documenting what you eat outside of your home is going to be challenging.

Making Volumetrics work for you

As with any diet, the key to success on the Volumetrics diet is following the plan in good faith and adjusting it where necessary to fit your lifestyle.

What do we mean by good faith? Zumpano puts it best, explaining, "We are in a hacking world, and it's OK to hack your diet once in a while. But if you do it on a regular basis, you're not going to reap the benefits as intended."

Think about it as embracing the spirit of the diet, not the letter of it. Yes, nuts and fast food are in the same category, but we all know that a handful of almonds is a better choice than a handful of pretzels. Unlike plans that integrate a peer-support system of some kind, you're only accountable to yourself on the Volumetrics diet.

While the freedom that comes with the Volumetrics diet may tempt some people to try and game the system, it also makes it adaptable to your needs. That, in turn, makes it sustainable.

How do you adjust the Volumetrics diet to fit your goals and lifestyle?

Here are a few examples:
• Let's say you're trying to get healthy, but don't actually need to lose weight. You could adjust the number of calories you're taking in each day, while maintaining the ratios prescribed in the diet. You could also ignore calories altogether and focus exclusively on nutrition.
• Let's say you do want to lose weight, but calorie counting puts you in a less-than-healthy head space. Don't do it! Try recording the number of foods you eat from each of the four categories instead, or make a healthy-eating checklist for yourself.
• Let's say you can't exercise for 30 minutes a day. Then do what you can! Five minutes of stretching or taking the stairs instead of the elevator is 100% better than doing nothing. Set realistic and attainable goals that fit your current health and fitness level. Once you crush it, you can set your sights higher.

Is the Volumetrics diet right for you?

Like all diet plans, your mileage may vary when it comes to Volumetrics. If you're trying to decide whether or not to adopt this approach to eating, the following questions may prove helpful:
• Are you looking for a quick fix or a lifestyle change? The Volumetrics plan is about long-term healthy eating, not short-term weight loss. If you just need to drop a couple of extra pounds, this probably isn't the best choice.

• Are you a decent cook? Do you consider assembling a salad cooking? Does the fire alarm serve as the soundtrack for your culinary adventures? Or is a food delivery service your most-used app? If your answer to any of these questions is "yes," you may want to opt for a less cooking-intensive diet.

• Where do you live and what's your budget? On the one hand, the Volumetrics diet doesn't require you to purchase branded specialty foods, which can be prohibitively expensive. On the other hand, not all people have equal access to good quality fruits and vegetables, and inflation has made healthy food even less accessible than it used to be. Look carefully at what you're spending your grocery budget on right now, and see where you can make healthy substitutions.

• Do you have any gastrointestinal issues? If you have a digestive disorder like irritable bowel syndrome (IBS), you may find that certain otherwise-healthy foods exacerbate your symptoms. You can still follow the Volumetrics diet, but opt for low-FODMAP foods, which are less likely to trigger a flare. Your tummy will thank you.

Some diets, like the DASH diet or the diabetes diet, are designed to address specific health concerns. The Volumetrics diet isn't, so you're unlikely to hear about it from your physician unless you ask about it specifically. Before making any radical nutritional changes, do some additional research, and have a conversation with a doctor or dietitian.

Volumetrics Diet Sample Menu Plan

We have prepared a sample volumetrics meal plan for you which is prepared for your guidance and which you can adjust within the diet plan you are currently following as per your weight loss needs. It is worth noting that you must amend the given sample plan according to your own diet plan and calorie requirement.

Monday
Breakfast
• Banana Yogurt Pots: 225g Greek yogurt, 2 sliced bananas, 15g walnuts chopped
Lunch
• Cannellini Bean Salad: 3 cups Cannellini beans, 30g cherry tomatoes, ½ red onion, ½ Tbsp. red wine vinegar, and a small bunch of basil
Dinner
• Quick Moussaka: 1 Tbsp. olive oil, ½ onion, 1 garlic clove, 250g lean beef, 200g chopped tomatoes, 1 tsp. grounded cinnamon, 200g chickpeas, 100g feta cheese, mint, and brown bread
Protein – 61g
Carbs – 132g
Fat – 34g
Total Calories per Day: 1,078 kcal

Tuesday
Breakfast
• Tomato and Watermelon Salad: 1 Tbsp. olive oil, 1 Tbsp. red wine vinegar, ¼ tsp. chili flakes, 1 Tbsp. chopped mint, 120g tomatoes, ½ watermelon, 50g feta cheese
Lunch

• Edgy Veggie Wraps: 100g cherry tomatoes, 1 cucumber, 6 Kalamata olives, 2 large whole-wheat tortilla wraps, 50g feta cheese, 2 Tbsp. hummus
Dinner
• Spicy Tomato Baked Eggs: 1 Tbsp. olive oil, 2 red onions, 1 red chili,1 garlic clove, 800g cherry tomatoes, 4 eggs, chopped coriander, and brown bread
Protein – 35g
Carbs – 97g
Fat – 41g
Total Calories per Day: 897 Kcal

Wednesday
Breakfast
• Blueberry Oats Bowl: 60g porridge oats, 160g Greek yogurt, 175g blueberries, 1 tsp. honey
Lunch
• Carrot, Orange and Avocado Salad: 1 orange, 2 carrots, 35g arugula, 1 avocado, 1 tbsp. olive oil
Dinner
• Salmon with Potatoes and Corn Salad: 200g baby new tomatoes, 1 sweetcorn cob, 2 skinless salmon filets, 60g tomatoes, 1 tbsp. red wine vinegar, 1 tbsp. olive oil, 1 tbsp. capers, a bunch of spring onions and basil leaves
Protein – 61g
Carbs – 78g
Fat – 38g
Total Calories per Day: 898 Kcal

Thursday
Breakfast
• Banana Yogurt Pots: 225g Greek yogurt, 2 sliced bananas, 15g walnuts chopped

Lunch
• Mixed Bean Salad: 145g cups jar artichoke heart, ½ tbsp.
sun-dried tomatoes, ½ tsp. red wine vinegar, 200g
cannellini beans, 150g tomatoes, 2 spring onions, 100g feta
cheese, and a handful of Kalamata olives
Dinner
• Spiced Carrot and Lentil Soup: 1 tsp. cumin seeds, 1 tbsp.
olive oil, 300g carrots, 70g red lentils, 500ml vegetable
stock, 60ml milk, Greek yogurt
Protein – 36g
Carbs – 88g
Fat – 26g
Total Calories per Day: 730 Kcal

Friday
Breakfast
• Tomato and Watermelon Salad: 1 Tbsp. olive oil, 1 Tbsp.
red wine vinegar, ¼ tsp. chilli flakes, 1 Tbsp. chopped
mint, 120g tomatoes, ½ watermelon, 50g feta cheese
Lunch
• Panzanella Salad: 400g tomatoes, 1 garlic clove, 1 tbsp.
capers, 1 ripe avocado, 1 small red onion, 2 slices of brown
bread, 2 tbsp. olive oil, 1 tbsp. red wine vinegar, a handful
of basil leaves
Dinner
• Med Chicken, Quinoa and Greek Salad: 100g quinoa, ½
red chilli, 2 chicken breasts, 1 garlic clove, 150g tomatoes,
1 tbsp. olive oil, ½ red onion, 50g feta cheese, a small
bunch of mint leaves, lemon zest
Protein – 47g
Carbs – 107g
Fat – 63g
Total Calories per Day: 1,247 Kcal

Saturday
Breakfast
• Blueberry Oats Bowl: 60g porridge oats, 160g Greek yogurt, 175g blueberries, 1 tsp. honey
Lunch
• Quinoa and Stir-Fried Veg: 100g quinoa, 3 tbsp. olive oil, 1 garlic clove,2 carrots, 150g leek, 1 broccoli head, 50g tomatoes, 100ml vegetable stock, 1 tsp. tomato puree, ½ lemon juice
Dinner
• Grilled Vegetables with Bean Mash: 1 pepper, 1 aubergine, 2 courgettes, 2 tbsp. olive oil, 400g haricot beans, 1 garlic clove, 100ml vegetable stock, 1 tbsp. chopped coriander
Protein – 43g
Carbs – 127g
Fat – 45g
Total Calories per Day: 1,085 Kcal

Sunday
Breakfast
• Banana Yogurt Pots: 225g Greek yogurt, 2 sliced bananas, 15g walnuts chopped
Lunch
• Moroccan Chickpea Soup: 1 tbsp. olive oil, ½ medium onion,1 celery stick, 1 tsp. ground cumin, 300ml vegetable stock, 200g chopped tomatoes, 200g chickpeas, 50g frozen broad beans, ½ lemon zest, coriander
Dinner
• Spicy Mediterranean Beet Salad: 8 raw baby beetroots, ½ tbsp. sumac, ½ tbsp. cumin, 400g chickpeas, 2 tbsp. olive oil, ½ tsp. lemon zest, ½ tsp. lemon juice, 200g Greek yogurt, 1 tbsp. harissa paste, 1 tsp. chilli flakes, mint leaves

Protein – 52g
Carbs – 153g
Fat – 38g
Total Calories per Day: 1,282 Kcal

Summary
The 7-day volumetric diet meal plan for weight loss is a balanced and healthy eating plan that can help you shed unwanted pounds. The key to success with this plan is to make sure you're getting enough volume of food each day and the right mix of nutrients. This meal plan provides plenty of both and can be easily customized to your own preferences and calorie needs. With a little bit of prep work, the 7-day volumetric diet meal plan can help you reach your weight loss goals in a sustainable and delicious way!

The Ultimate Volumetrics diet recipes

Italian Layered Pudding

Difficulty: Easy
Preparation: 25 min

Ingredients

1. ⅜ cup warm, strong, black coffee
2. 6 tbsps coffee liqueur (or brandy)
3. 20 ladyfinger
4. 1 ⅛ cups mascarpone
5. 4 eggs (separated)
6. 4 tbsps caster sugar
7. 1 tbsp cocoa powder

Preparation steps
1. Mix the coffee with 2 tablespoons coffee liqueur or brandy. Dip the sponge fingers in the mixture and lay in a serving dish. Pour over any remaining coffee mixture.
2. Beat together the mascarpone, egg yolks, sugar and remaining liqueur or brandy.
3. Whisk the egg whites until stiff, but not dry and gently fold into the mascarpone mixture until blended. Spoon over the sponge fingers.
4. Sift the cocoa over the top. Chill for at least 2 hours before serving.

VEGAN BARLEY SOUP (VOLUMETRICS)

Ready In: 40mins
Ingredients: 13
Yields: 5 cups
Serves: 4

INGREDIENTS
• 1⁄2 cup chopped onion
• 1⁄4 cup chopped celery
• 1 tablespoon chopped parsley
• 1⁄2 teaspoon chopped garlic
• 3 1⁄2 cups vegetable broth
• 1 1⁄2 cups canned diced tomatoes, with liquid
• 1⁄4 cup pearl barley
• 1⁄4 teaspoon salt ground black pepper
• 1⁄4 teaspoon dried oregano
• 1⁄4 teaspoon dried thyme
• 1 bay leaf
• 2 cups chopped mushrooms

DIRECTIONS
1. Spray a large pot with cooking spray and place over medium-high heat until hot. Add the onion, celery, parsley, and garlic and cook, atirrring frequently, 4 minutes.
2. Add the broth through the bay leaf and bring to a simmer. Cover and simmer, stirring occasionally, for 20 minutes.
3. Add the mushrooms and simmer another 20 minutes.
4. Remove and discard bay leaf before serving.

Sautéed Spicy Cabbage

PREP TIME: 10 minutes
COOK TIME: 25 minutes
TOTAL TIME: 35minutes
COURSE: Side Dish

INGREDIENTS
• 1 small white cabbage (about 10 cups shredded)
• 1 large onion
• 2 tbsp olive oil
• 1 cup water, divided
• 2 tsp salt
• 1 tsp thyme (you can omit this or sub in any spice of choice)
• 1 cup apple cider vinegar
• 1 tbsp hot sauce (change amount according to your taste)
• 1 tbsp chopped parsley

INSTRUCTIONS
• With a sharp knife (or a mandolin), thinly slice your cabbage and onion.
• In a cast iron pan (you can use any pan but cast iron gives a nice smokiness to it!), add in the olive oil and heat over high heat until very hot.
• Add onion and cabbage and stir to coat in oil; cook on high heat for about 5 minutes (the bottom should start to caramelize)
• Stir well and add 1/2 cup of water; stir again and cook for 3 minutes.
• Add the rest of the water and cook for another 5 minutes, stirring as the cabbage softens

• Add 2 tsp salt and spices, then add the apple cider vinegar and hot sauce; stir well and cook for an additional 10 minutes on medium low (stirring) until cabbage is soft and to your liking.
• Stir in the parsely and serve as a side dish.

VOLUMETRICS FAJITA BREAKFAST BURRITO

Ready In: 20mins
Ingredients: 9
Yields: 1 recipe
Serves: 4

INGREDIENTS
• 2 medium bell peppers, seeded and chopped
• 1 medium red onion, peeled and chopped
• 8 large eggs
• 1/3 cup reduced-fat monterey jack and cheddar cheese blend
• salt and pepper
• 4 whole wheat tortillas
• 1/4 cup reduced-fat sour cream
• 1 avocado, split, pitted, peeled and sliced
• 1/4 cup salsa

DIRECTIONS
1. Spray a large skillet with cooking spray and place over medium heat. Cook the peppers and onion, stirring

occasionally, until soft, about 5 minutes. Transfer the mixture to a bowl.

2. Whisk the eggs in a seperate medium bowl. Spray the skillet again with cooking spray. Scramble in the skillet over medium heat until fully cooked. Stir in the peppers and onion mixture and cheese, and season with salt and pepper to taste. Remove from the heat.

3. Spread each whole-wheat tortilla with 1 tablespoon of sour cream down the center and top with one-quarter of the avocado slices. Place one-quarter of the egg mixture on each tortilla, fold over the side edges, and roll into a burrito. Top each with 1 tablespoon of salsa.

Shakshuka with Tomatoes and Zucchini

Difficulty: Moderate
Preparation: 35 min
Calories: 522 calories

Ingredients
1. 2 small zucchini
2. 1 bunch scallions
3. 2 garlic cloves
4. 3 tbsps olive oil
5. 1 tsp cumin
6. 14 ozs tomatoes
7. 1 pinch cayenne pepper (or chili flakes)
8. salt peppers
9. 4 eggs
10. 3 ½ ozs feta
11. 2 stalks parsley

Preparation steps
1. Clean and wash the zucchini and spring onions and cut into slices or rings. Peel and chop the garlic.
2. Heat oil in a pan and fry spring onions, zucchini, garlic and cumin for about 5-6 minutes at medium heat. Add tomato pieces, cayenne pepper, salt and pepper. Simmer for another 6-7 minutes at medium heat.
3. Form four small hollows in the tomato mixture. Slide the eggs evenly into the hollows. Let the eggs set for 15-20 minutes, covering them with a lid. Shortly before cooking, crumble the cheese, pour over the eggs and allow to melt slightly. Wash the parsley, shake dry, chop and sprinkle the parsley over the shakshuka.

Potato Soup with Coconut Milk

Difficulty: Easy
Preparation: 25 min
Calories: 380 calories

Ingredients
1. 5 stalks celery
2. 2 large potatoes
3. 1 onion
4. 1 pc ginger
5. 2 tbsps coconut oil
6. 2 cups vegetable broth
7. 2 carrots
8. salt
9. peppers
10. ½ tsp ground turmeric
11. ½ cup coconut milk

12. 1 pinch cayenne pepper

Preparation steps
1. Clean and peel the celery, potatoes, onion and ginger and cut everything into small pieces. Cut 3 TBSP celery into cubes and put aside.
2. Heat 1 tablespoon of oil in a pot. First fry the onion and ginger until translucent, then add the vegetables and sauté. Add the stock and cook over medium heat for about 15 minutes until soft.
3. At the same time peel carrots and cut into small cubes. Heat 1 tablespoon of oil in a pan and fry the carrot and celery cubes for 7 minutes. Season with salt, pepper and turmeric.
4. Puree the soup with the coconut milk using a hand blender. Season to taste with salt, pepper and cayenne pepper. Pour the vegetable cubes over the soup and serve.

SWEET AND SOUR CHICKEN (LOW FAT AND VOLUMETRIC)

Ready In: 30mins
Ingredients: 12
Serves: 6

INGREDIENTS
• 1 tablespoon oil 6 boneless skinless chicken breast halves (chopped in chunks)
• 2 bell peppers (any color, chopped in chunks)
• 1 onion (large, chopped in chunks)
• 1 cup vinegar

- 1/2 teaspoon salt
- 1/2 cup orange juice
- 1/2 cup pineapple juice (from a can of pineapple chunks)
- 6 ounces tomato paste (1 can)
- 2 tablespoons cornstarch (dissolved in cold water)
- 1/3 cup Splenda sugar substitute
- 1 cup pineapple chunk

DIRECTIONS
1. Heat oil in a non-stick pan or wok.
2. Cook chicken until no longer pink. Remove chicken, saving the liquid in the pan.
3. Add the peppers and onions to the liquid in the pan and heat until cooked. I like my peppers and onions crunchy, so I don't overcook.
4. Once cooked, drain and set aside.
5. While chicken and peppers are cooking, prepare the sauce.
6. To make sauce: place vinegar, salt, juices and tomato paste in a pot.
7. Heat on medium and simmer for 10 minutes.
8. Combine cornstarch with a small amount of water.
9. Add cornstarch/water mixture to the sauce, stirring to remove any lumps.
10. Add splenda and pineapple chunks.
11. Continue to heat for another couple of minutes to heat pineapple chunks.
12. Serving ideas: Either combine the sauce with the cooked chicken mixture, or serve the sauce on the side. Present with steamed rice.

Susan's Dirty Little Secret Soup

Prep Time: 10 minutes
Cook Time: 30 minutes
Total Time: 40 minutes
Servings 8

Ingredients
• 5-6 cups vegetable broth I use Imagine No-Chicken
• 1 16- ounce can diced tomatoes
• 2 16- ounce cans beans rinsed and drained (I usually use 1 Great Northern and 1 Kidney Bean)
• 2 1- pound bags of frozen vegetables (my favorites are California Blend [cauliflower, broccoli, and carrots] and Italian Blend [zucchini, Italian green beans, broccoli, red pepper])
• 4 cloves minced garlic
• 1 teaspoon basil
• 1/2 teaspoons oregano
• 1/2 teaspoon thyme
• a shake or two of hot pepper sauce (Tabasco)
• black pepper and salt to taste
• 1/2 cup small pasta OR 2 cups diced potatoes OR 1 cup frozen corn or other starchy vegetable OR 1/2 cup of quick-cooking grain (buckwheat, pearled barley, millet, or quinoa or cooked rice OPTIONAL

Instructions
• Put 5 cups of vegetable broth and all remaining ingredients into a large pot. Bring to a boil, reduce heat, and simmer until vegetables are done, about 20-30 minutes.

If the soup seems too thick, add more broth. Taste and adjust seasonings before serving.
• This can also be made with 2 pounds of whatever fresh vegetables you have in the house.

CANNELLINI BEAN SOUP (VOLUMETRICS)

Ready In: 30mins
Ingredients: 14
Yields: 6 cups
Serves: 4

INGREDIENTS
• 1 teaspoon olive oil
• 1 cup chopped onion
• 1 1/2 teaspoons chopped garlic
• 1 cup water
• 2 cups cored died tomatoes
• 2 cups canned cannellini beans, drained and rinsed
• 1 cup diced zucchini
• 1/2 cup frozen peas, thawed
• 1 cup thinly sliced carrot
• 1 tablespoon chopped flat leaf parsley
• 3/4 teaspoon dried thyme
• fresh ground black pepper
• 2 cups vegetable broth
• 4 tablespoons parmesan cheese

DIRECTIONS
1. Lightly spray a 4 to 5 quart pot with cooking spray and place over medium heat. Add the oil, onion, and garlic and cook 5 minutes, stirring frequently.
2. Stir in remaining ingredients (except cheese) and bring to a simmer, stirring occasionally. Simmer 10 minutes, stirring occasionally. Sprinkle with Parmesan when serving.

WEIGHT LOSS WONDER SOUP

INGREDIENTS
• 1/2 teaspoon olive oil, optional
• 4 large onions, finely chopped (6-8 coups)
• 2 green bell pepper, diced (2-3 cups)
• 3 large tomatoes, roughly chopped (3-4 cups)
• 1 bunch celery, diced (3-4 cups)
• 1 small cabbage, chopped (10-12 cups)
• 3 cup water, or up to 5 cups for a more watery soup

INSTRUCTIONS
1. Start off by cutting up all the vegetables and separating them into three large bowls: onion and green pepper in the first bowl, tomatoes and celery in the second bowl, and cabbage in the last bowl.
2. In a large skillet, heat olive oil over medium-high heat. Add onions and green peppers to pan, tossing to coat. Sautee veggies until water has cooked out and onions begin to brown. The length of time this takes will depend on your cooking unit and the size of your pan, but for me, it took about 35 minutes. Turn the veggies every 3 to 5 minutes

while cooking to prevent sticking and to check the color. Once cooked, remove pan from heat.

3. In a 12 quart stockpot, add the cabbage and water. Next, add the tomatoes and celery. Finish by adding the cooked onions and green peppers on top. Ingredients will likely be to be brim of the pot - this is okay. Do not stir soup yet.

4. Heat the soup over medium-high until water begins to boil. By this point, the veggies should have cooked down some, giving you room to stir. Once veggies are mixed, reduce heat so soup is simmering and cook for 50-60 minutes, stirring occasionally.

5. If desired, serve soup immediately. Store excess soup in a sealed container in the refrigerator for up to 5 days.

Warm Vegetable Salad

Ingredients

1. 2 small zucchini (125 grams)
2. ½ cauliflower (300 grams)
3. 3 carrots (each approximately 85 grams)
4. ½ small hokkaido pumpkin (400 grams)
5. 1 red onion
6. 1 garlic clove
7. 250 grams chickpeas (canned, drained)
8. ½ baguette (about 125 grams)
9. 100 grams goat cheese
10. 4 sprigs thyme
11. 3 tbsps olive oil
12. 125 milliliters vegetable broth
13. 1 lemon
14. salt

15. peppers
16. 1 tsp black cumin seeds

Kitchen utensils
1. 1 cutting board, 1 small knife, 1 peeler, 1 tablespoon, 1 large knife, 1 sieve, 1 serrated knife, 1 knife, 1 baking sheet, 1 wide pot (with lid), 1 wooden spoon, 1 measuring cups, 1 large bowl, 1 citrus juicer, 1 salad server

Preparation steps
1. Rinse zucchini, cut in half lengthwise and cut into 1 cm (approximately 1/2-inch) slices. Trim cauliflower, rinse and divide into florets.
2. Rinse and peel carrots. Cut into thin slices.
3. Remove pumpkin seeds with a spoon. Rinse and cut flesh into 1 cm (approximately 1/2-inch) cubes.
4. Peel onion and garlic. Cut onion into thin strips and finely dice garlic
5. Drain the chickpeas and rinse under water until water runs clear. Drain well.
6. Cut baguette into 12 slices, spread with goat cheese and place on a baking sheet
7. Rinse thyme, shake dry, pluck leaves, sprinkle over the goat cheese and press gently, adhering to cheese.
8. Heat 1 tablespoon of oil in a large pot. Add onion, garlic, carrots, pumpkin and cauliflower. Sauté for 2 minutes, while stirring constantly.
9. Pour in broth, cover and simmer over medium heat about 5 minutes.
10. Add zucchini and chickpeas and continue to cook for 5 minutes. Transfer to a large bowl.
11. Cut lemon in half and squeeze juice over vegetables. Drizzle with the remaining oil and season with salt and

pepper. Mix well. Sprinkle in cumin seeds. Place baguette slices under a preheated broiler or oven at 250°C (approximately 475°F) until the cheese browns, about 2 minutes. Serve baguette slices with the warm vegetable salad.

Volumetrics Red White and Blue Trifle

1. Makes 15 servings of 1 cup each.
2. Number of Servings: 15

INGREDIENTS
1. 1 15-oz carton low-fat ricotta cheese
2. 1 6-oz carton fat-free or low-fat lemon or vanilla yogurt
3. 1/2 cup powdered sugar
4. 2 tsp. vanilla extract
5. 1 10-inch round angel food cake, cut into 1-inch cubes
6. 1 medium banana
7. 2 tsp. lemon juice
8. 2 c. frozen, thawed unsweetened wild blueberries
9. 2 c. fresh blackberries
10. 2 c. fresh sliced strawberries
11. 1 1/2 cups frozen fat-free whipped topping, thawed

DIRECTIONS
1. Combine the ricotta, yogurt, powdered sugar and vanilla in an electric blender, and process until smooth. Set aside.
2. Layer one-third of the cake cubes in the bottom of a large trifle bowl or deep serving bowl. Spoon one-third of the ricotta mixture evenly over the cake cubes.
3. Peel and slice the banana, and toss the slices with lemon juice.

4. Layer one-third of the banana and berries on top. Repeat with layers of cake, ricotta mixture, and fruit twice. Spread the whipped topping over the top layer of fruit. Cover and refrigerate at least 2 hours before serving.

MINESTRONE (VOLUMETRICS)

Ready In: 1hr
Ingredients: 13
Yields: 8 cups
Serves: 8

INGREDIENTS
• 2 teaspoons olive oil
• 1 cup chopped onion
• 1 cup shredded carrot
• 1 cup water
• 1 1/2 cups low-sodium vegetable juice (V8)
• 3 cups vegetable broth
• 1 1/4 cups cored diced tomatoes
• 3/4 teaspoon dried thyme
• 1 teaspoon dried oregano
• black pepper
• 3/4 cup small whole wheat pasta, cooked separately (shells or other shape)
• 1 cup canned cannellini beans, rinsed and drained
• 3 cups shredded spinach

DIRECTIONS

1. Heat the oil in a 4 to 5 quart pan over medium heat. Add onions and carrots and cook 5 minutes, stirring occasionally.

2. Add the water, juice, broth, tomatoes, thyme, oregano, and pepper. Bring the soup to a boil, reduce the heat, and simmer, covered, for 30 minutes.

3. Add the cooked pasta, beans, and spinach and cook on medium-low until spinach wilts.

BARLEY-STUFFED ACORN SQUASH (VOLUMETRICS)

Ready In: 1hr 10mins
Ingredients: 10
Serves: 4

Ingredients

INGREDIENTS
UNITS: US
• 2 acorn squash, halved and seeded
• 1 1/2 cups cooked barley
• 1/2 cup chopped scallion
• 1/2 cup finely chopped celery
• 2 tablespoons toasted pine nuts
• 2 tablespoons chopped fresh marjoram
• 2 teaspoons olive oil
• 1/2 teaspoon salt
• 1/4 teaspoon fresh ground black pepper
• 1 teaspoon paprika

DIRECTIONS

1. Preheat oven to 350 Fahrenheit. Coat a baking sheet with cooking spray.
2. Place the squash, cut sides up, on the baking sheet and bake 25 minutes.
3. Combine remaining ingredients (except paprika) in a medium bowl. Divide this mixture amongst the squash cavities. Sprinkle with paprika and bake 20 to 25 minutes, or until squash is tender.

RASPBERRY-APPLE CRUMBLE (VOLUMETRIC)

Ready In: 1hr 15mins
Ingredients: 10
Yields: 6 one cup servings
Serves: 6

INGREDIENTS
• 6 medium tart apples (such as Granny Smith)
• 1/3 cup orange juice
• 1/3 cup water
• 3 tablespoons raspberry jam (I use light jam)
• 1/3 cup oatmeal
• 3 tablespoons flour
• 3 tablespoons brown sugar (I use Splenda brown sugar blend)
• 1 1/2 teaspoons cinnamon
• 1 pinch salt
• 1 1/2 tablespoons reduced-calorie margarine (Melted)

DIRECTIONS
1. Preheat oven to 350 degrees.
2. Combine juice, water, and jam.
3. Core apples and slice thinly. (I usually slice in quarters and then slice each quarter into 4 more slices for a total of 16 per apple).
4. As you slice each apple, place in juice mixture and stir to cover apples so they won't turn brown.
5. Pour mixture into an 8x8 pan.
6. Combine remaining dry ingredients and stir to mix well, then add melted margarine. Stir again to mix. Mixture will be crumbly.
7. Sprinkle oat mixture over apple mixture.
8. Bake 1 hour or until apples are tender.
9. Serve hot or room temperature, on its own or with low fat ice cream. Keeps very well in the fridge (if there is any left over) and is delicious cold the next day.
10. Tip: prepare in advance and place in oven at the start of your meal for a hot dessert.

GREAT AMERICAN VOLUMETRIC BURGER

Ready In: 55mins
Ingredients: 12
Yields: 4 patties
Serves: 4

INGREDIENTS
UNITS: US
• 1/3 cup bulgur, uncooked

- 1/2 cup boiling water
- 2 teaspoons olive oil
- 1 cup red onion, minced
- 1/2 teaspoon sugar
- 1 teaspoon balsamic vinegar
- 3/4 lb extra lean ground beef or 3/4 lb turkey
- 1 large garlic clove
- 3/4 cup finely grated carrot, lightly packed
- 2 teaspoons Worcestershire sauce
- 1/2 teaspoon salt
- 1/2 teaspoon fresh ground pepp

DIRECTIONS

1. Stir together the bulgur and 1/2 cup boiling water in a small bowl; let stand 30 minutes or until water is absorbed and bulgur is tender.

2. Meanwhile, in a nonstick skillet, heat the olive oil over medium heat. Add the onion and sugar; saute until the onion is lightly browned, about 10 minutes. Stir in the vinegar; saute about 20 seconds, stirring until vinegar evaporates. Remove the skillet from the heat.

3. In a small bowl, mix the plumped bulgur, onion mixture, beef, carrot, garlic, Worcestershire sauce, salt and pepper.

4. Shape into 3/4-thick patties.

5. Grill or broil the burger patties on a rack sprayed with vegetable cooking spray until browned and cooked, about 5 minutes per side.

6. Serve on bun with desired condiments.

Two-fruit Crumble Cups

Difficulty: Easy
Preparation: 45 min

Ingredients
1. 1 cup cranberry (lightly crushed with a fork)
2. 2 pear (peeled, cored and roughly chopped)
3. 1 tsp cinnamon
4. 2 tbsps honey
5. ¼ cup butter
6. ⅓ cup brown sugar
7. ⅓ cup flour
8. 2 tbsps oatmeal
9. whipped cream (to serve)

Preparation steps
1. Heat the oven to 200°C (180° fan) 400°F, gas 6.
2. Mix together the cranberries, chopped pears and cinnamon, divide between 4 individual ovenproof serving dishes and drizzle with the honey.
3. Rub together the butter, sugar and flour until the mixture resembles breadcrumbs then stir in the oatmeal. Scatter the mixture over the top of the dishes and bake in the oven for 15 - 20 minutes. Srve with the whipped cream.

CURRIED CAULIFLOWER SOUP (VOLUMETRICS)

Ready In: 30mins
Ingredients: 8
Yields:6
Serves: 4

INGREDIENTS
- 1 tablespoon olive oil
- 1 1/2 cups halved and sliced onions
- 1 teaspoon curry powder
- 2 cups vegetable broth
- 2 cups water
- 4 cups chopped cauliflower florets
- 1/2 teaspoon salt
- 2 cups shredded zucchini

DIRECTIONS
1. Heat the oil in a 4 to 5 quart pot over medium heat. Add the onions and curry powder, cover, and cook 4 minutes, stirring occasionally.
2. Add the broth, water, cauliflower, and salt to the pot.Bring to a simmer, stirring occasionally, then cover and simmer 15 minutes, stirring occasionally.
3. Puree the soup in a blender or food processor and return to the pot.
4. Reserve 2 tablespoons of the zucchini and stir the rest into the soup and reheat.
5. Ladle the soup into 4 soup bowls and garnish with the reserves zucchini.

Vegetable Soup

Difficulty: Easy
Preparation: 30 min
Calories: 78 calories

Ingredients
1. 8 ozs potatoes
2. 2 small carrots
3. 3 zucchini
4. 1 cup water
5. 2 cups vegetable broth
6. ½ bunch parsley
7. salt
8. peppers

Preparation steps
1. Peel, rinse and slice the potatoes. Rinse and slice the carrots. Rinse and slice the summer squash.
2. Heat the oil in a pan and saute the vegetables for 5 minutes. Pour in the water and vegetable broth. Simmer over low heat for 12 minutes. Season with salt and pepper. Rinse the parsley and sprinkle on the soup. Serve hot.

CREAMY BROCCOLI SOUP (VOLUMETRICS)

Ready In: 30mins
Ingredients: 9
Yields: 4 cups
Serves: 4

INGREDIENTS
• 2 tablespoons butter
• 3/4 cup chopped onion
• 2 tablespoons all-purpose flour
• 1 teaspoon dry mustard white pepper
• 2 cups nonfat milk
• 2 cups chicken stock (use vegetable broth for vegan version)
• 4 cups chopped broccoli florets
• 1 1/2 - 2 teaspoons fresh tarragon

DIRECTIONS
1. Melt the butter in a 4 to 5 quart pan over medium heat. Add the onions and sweat them, stirring occasionally, 5 minutes.
2. Raise the heat to medium-high and stir in the flour, mustard, and pepper and cook 2 minutes. Reduce heat to medium, add the milk and stock and cook, stirring frequently, 8 minutes. Add the broccoli and simmer 6 minutes, stirring frequently. Remove from heat, puree 2 cups of soup in a blender, and return pureed soup to pot. Reheat, stirring occasionally, about 2 minutes.

Brown Rice Cereal with Mango and Cardamom

Difficulty: Easy
Preparation: 25 Min Ready in 1hr 10 min
calories: 269 calories

Ingredients
1. 6 ozs brown rice
2. 1 oz dried mangoes

3. 2 tbsps banana chip
4. 2 cups
5. 2 sprigs lemon balm
6. 1 tbsp maple syrup
7. 1 pinch ground cardamom
8. 1 tsp ground cinnamon
9. 1 tbsp coconut flakes

Kitchen utensils
1. 1 pot (with lid), 1 measuring cups, 1 cutting board, 1 large knife, 1 small knife, 1 tablespoon, 1 teaspoon, 1 wooden spoon, 1 lid

Preparation steps
1. Bring 2 cups of water to a boil in a pot and add the rice. Return to a boil, cover and cook over low heat until grains are tender and the water has been absorbed. (Rice can be prepared the day before and refrigerated, covered.)
2. Cut the dried mango into small pieces.
3. Coarsely chop the banana chips.
4. Add the milk to the cooked rice and bring to a boil. Cook over medium heat until creamy, stirring constantly, 5-6 minutes. Rinse the lemon balm, pat dry and pluck leaves.
5. Stir the mango, maple syrup, cardamom and cinnamon into the rice mixture. Cook over low heat, stirring, until heated through, about 3 minutes more. Pour porridge into bowls. Sprinkle with coconut and banana chips, garnish with lemon balm and serve.

Cocktail Penicillin (Penicillin)

Cooking Time: 3 min
Calories: 360

Ingredients
• 60 ml Black Label Whiskey
• 5-7 ml Talisker (or Laphroaig) whiskey
• 22-25 ml Fresh lemon (about half a lemon)
• 12 ml Honey syrup
• 12 ml Ginger syrup

Preparation
• Ginger syrup: grate the ginger, squeeze the juice, add a little sugar, evaporate.
• Honey syrup: 3 parts water, one part honey, evaporate.
• Add ice, ginger syrup, honey syrup, lemon juice and Black Label to the shaker.
• We shake, strain into a glass a chilled glass with ice.
• Pour Talisker on top (do not stir).
• Decorate with a slice of ginger.
• We drink without a straw.

CITRUS-GINGER DRESSING (VOLUMETRICS)

Ready In: 2mins
Ingredients: 8
Yields: 6 tbsp.
Serves: 4

INGREDIENTS
- 3 tablespoons lime juice
- 2 tablespoons water
- 2 tablespoons olive oil
- 1/2 teaspoon sugar
- 1 tablespoon minced fresh chives
- 1 teaspoon minced fresh ginger
- 1/4 teaspoon salt
- 1 pinch black pepper

DIRECTIONS
1. Combine all ingredients in a screw-top jar and shake vigorously until blended.

The Volumetrics Smoothie recipes

Avocado Spinach Smoothie Recipe

- PREP TIME: 10 mins
- TOTAL TIME: 10 mins
- COURSE: Beverage, Smoothie
- CUISINE: Global
- SERVINGS: 4 servingsCALORIES

INGREDIENTS

- 8 oz avocado (a large avocado)
- 2 oz spinach
- 8 oz banana
- 2 cups ice
- 1 cup milk
- 1/4 cup plain Greek yogurt
- 2 tbsp honey (optional)
- 6 mint leaves

INSTRUCTIONS
1. Put 2 cups of ice and scoop 8 oz avocado into the blender.
2. Add 8 oz banana, 1 cup milk, 1/4 cup Greek yogurt, honey (to your taste but no more than 2 tbsp), and 2 oz spinach.
3. Blend at high speed in 20 - 30 seconds until the mixture is smooth.
4. Transfer the smoothie into serving glasses.
5. Garnish with 6 mint leaves and serve immediately.

Orange Julius Smoothie

Prep Time: 5 minutes
Cook Time: 0 minutes
Total Time: 5 minutes
Servings: 2 servings
Course: Drink
Cuisine: American

Ingredients
• 1 cup ice cubes
• 1 medium frozen banana
• ½ cup plain greek yogurt
• ½ cup orange juice
• 2 teaspoons pure vanilla extract
• orange zest, from 1 orange
• 1 large orange, peeled and segmented
• 1 tablespoon ground flaxseed
• 1 teaspoon honey, maple syrup, or agave

Instructions
• Add ice, banana, yogurt, orange juice, vanilla, orange zest, oranges, ground flaxseed, and honey in a blender.
• Process until smooth, about 60 to 90 seconds.

Equipment
• Countertop Blender
• Decorative Paper Straws

Notes
1. Serving Size: 1 ¼ cup

High-Calorie Banana Smoothie for Weight Gain

PREP TIME: 3 minutes
BLEND TIME: 1 minute
TOTAL TIME: 4 minutes
COURSE: Smoothies
SERVINGS: 1 person
CALORIES: 989 kcal

EQUIPMENT
• 1 Blender
• 1 Spoon

INGREDIENTS
• 4 medium bananas (472 g)
• 6 oz 2% fat Greek yogurt (300 g)
• 1 oz roasted cashews (28 g)
• 1.8 oz oats (50 g)
• 10.2 fl oz water (300 ml)

INSTRUCTIONS
• Peel the bananas and break them so they will fit in the blender. 4 medium bananas
• Think whether the ingredients will fit inside your blender.In case you have a smaller blender, like the one we used for this recipe, split the ingredients into 2 or 3 equal portions, then follow the instructions for each portion separately.6 oz 2% fat Greek yogurt, 1 oz roasted cashews, 1.8 oz oats, 10.2 fl oz water, 4 medium bananas
• Add all the ingredients to the blender, making sure the water is at the bottom of the blender.If you have a blender with an ingredient recipient that needs to be turned upside

down when installed on the blender, always add the water lastly. This way, the blades will work smoothly instead of clogging in other ingredients.4 medium bananas, 6 oz 2% fat Greek yogurt, 1 oz roasted cashews, 1.8 oz oats, 10.2 fl oz water
• Blend the ingredients until the smoothie has a fine texture (about 30-60 seconds). If you have a weaker blender, you may want to mix the ingredients for longer than 1 minute. Nevertheless, to avoid overheating your blender, respect the blending time recommendation in your blender's manual.
• Pour the smoothie into a glass, or a shaker bottle, and serve.

NOTES
1. Besides helping you gain weight, this high-calorie banana smoothie has numerous other health benefits, such as raising potassium levels and helping you build muscle.

Green Mango Spinach Yogurt Smoothie

PREP TIME: 5 minutes
COOK TIME: 5 minutes
TOTAL TIME: 10 minutes
COURSE: Breakfast, Drinks
CUISINE: American
SERVINGS: 2 glasses
CALORIES: 123.94 kcal

EQUIPMENT
• Blender

INGREDIENTS
• ½ cup water
• 1 tablespoon chia seeds
• 1 cup baby spinach
• ½ cup Greek yogurt
• 1 orange
• ½ mango
• crushed ice optional

INSTRUCTIONS
• First, add water to the blender.
• Next, add chia seeds.
• Then, add baby spinach followed by low-fat Greek yogurt.
• Next, add in the orange slices and mango cubes
• Blend them all together to make a smooth and creamy smoothie.
• Pour the Super Healthy Mango Spinach Yogurt Power Smoothie into drinking glasses and serve immediately.

NOTES
1. I had some leftover raspberry which I crushed and used it as a garnish. It gave a nice contrast to the green smoothie. You can skip that if you don't have raspberries handy.
2. Since it's a low sugar green smoothie, there is no need to add any additional sugar or honey to the drink. You don't really miss the sugar as the smoothie is naturally sweet due to the ingredients used.
3. Add a dash of almond or cashew milk. The creamy smooth texture of these milk can mask some of the grassy taste caused by raw spinach and kale, making super greens taste less "green".

4. Feel free to add a protein powder of your choice along with chia seeds.

5. You can add frozen or fresh orange, mango, and spinach in here.

6. You can either add chia seeds without soaking and blend it along with the other ingredients or soak them and mix them in your smoothie before serving.

7. Add crushed ice while blending if you like your smoothie super chilled.

8. You need not strain this drink and can consume it as is. I do not like to strain my mango spinach smoothie.

9. To make it vegan, use any non-dairy yogurt instead of Greek yogurt.

4-Ingredient Banana Smoothie

Active time: 3 minutes
Total time: 3 minutes

Ingredients
1. Makes 1 Serving
2. ½ large, ripe banana, peeled, frozen, and cut into chunks
3. ½ cup unsweetened almond milk
4. ¼ cup plain 2-percent-fat Greek yogurt
5. 1 tablespoon almond butter

Preparation
1. Step 1 In a blender, puree all ingredients until smooth.
2. Step 2 Serve immediately, or refrigerate until ready to serve.

Apple Strawberry Smoothie for Weight Loss

PREP TIME: 5 minutes
TOTAL TIME: 5 minutes
COURSE: Snack
CUISINE: American
SERVINGS: 3 CALORIES

INGREDIENTS
• ½ cup unsweetened applesauce (frozen in ice cube trays)
• 1 cup chopped frozen strawberries
• 1½ cup milk
• ½ teaspoon vanilla extract
• ¼ teaspoon cardamom
• 2 tablespoons maple syrup (optional; use sugar-free syrup to keep it free of added sugars)

INSTRUCTIONS
• If you didn't freeze your applesauce in ice cube trays yet, make sure to do it before you start the recipe. Regular ice cube trays tend to hold 2 tablespoons in each compartment, so you will need 4 applesauce cubes for this recipe. The cubes are going to be much easier to blend than a ½ cup frozen block of applesauce!
• Put the frozen applesauce, strawberries, milk, vanilla, and cardamom in a food processor and blend until smooth. Taste it and add in the maple syrup or sugar free syrup if it's not sweet enough for you. Blend again.
• Pour the smoothie into tall glasses and serve with wide straws. Enjoy!

EQUIPMENT
• Food Processor

• Large-Width Straws

NOTES

1. This is a level 1 recipe (may help support fat loss). With about 100 calories per serving, this smoothie would blow most 100-calorie snack packs out of the water nutritionally. You've got the antioxidant-packed fruit, some protein and calcium from the milk, and a hydrating drink all in one. Take that, unsatisfying mini-bag containing 100 calories of low-quality cookies!.
2. The combination of apples and strawberries is flavorful and provides a lot of fluid volume and fiber. This smoothie is a great way to slip more fruit into breakfast, or incorporate it into a snack.
3. Don't forget that any modifications you make to the recipe will change the nutrition information. Many unsweetened plant milks are lower calorie than dairy milk. However, they don't get as airy when you whip them, so this recipe may only make 2 servings instead of 3.
4. Using the maple syrup in this recipe adds 35 calories per serving. Use a sugar free syrup instead if you want to cut back on calories and added sugar.

Green Protein Smoothie

PREP TIME: 5 minutes
TOTAL TIME: 5 minutes
SERVINGS: 1

Ingredients
• 1 frozen banana

• 1 scoop vanilla protein powder
• 1 cup cold unsweetened vanilla almond milk, or other milk
• 2 cups baby spinach, loosely packed
• 1 Tablespoon chia seeds

Instructions
• Place all ingredients into a high-powered blender and blend until smooth.

Notes
• What to use instead of protein powder: If you don't have protein powder on hand, you can add protein in a variety of ways. You can mix in Greek yogurt, nuts, nut butter or seeds. I tried this smoothie with Greek yogurt instead of protein powder and it was very spinachy so I'd recommend using only 1 cup spinach if using yogurt as the protein. If you add nuts or seeds, I recommend adding about 2 Tablespoons total.
• What to swap the banana with: You can replace the frozen banana with ice or frozen milk ice cubes (about 1 cup), frozen cauliflower rice (start with 1/4 cup), frozen zucchini or other frozen fruit like mangos or peaches.

Healthy Salted Caramel Smoothie Recipe | No Sugar Added!

• Prep Time: 5 mins
• Cook Time: 5 mins
• Total Time: 10 mins
• Yield: 1

Ingredients
- 1 1/2 frozen bananas
- 1 cup non-dairy milk of choice
- 4 large dates, pitted (or use 5 small)
- 1 tablespoon ground flaxseed, optional
- 1 tablespoon nut butter, optional
- 1/8 teaspoon kosher salt

Instructions
1. Place bananas, milk, dates, flaxseed (if using), nut butter (if using), and salt in a blender.
2. Cover and blend until ingredients are processed and smooth, about 1-2 minutes. Optional: garnish with a sprinkle of ground flaxseed and a date*.
3. Enjoy!

Notes
1. To garnish with the date, remove the pit and put a small cut into the bottom end of the date, about halfway through the date (vertical). Slide the date onto the edge of the cup.

Peach mango bliss smoothie (paleo & vegan)

- Total Time: 5 minutes
- Yield: 2 (large) or 4 (small)

INGREDIENTS
- 1 heaping cup frozen peach slices
- 1 heaping cup frozen mango slices
- 1/2 frozen banana (about 1/2 cup)
- 3/4–1 cup orange juice (more or less, to taste)
- 3/4–1 cup water (as needed, to blend)

• Optional: 1 scoop collagen powder, 1-2 Tbsp chia seeds, or 1 cup greens

INSTRUCTIONS
• Add all ingredients to a blender and puree until smooth, adding more orange juice or water as needed.

NOTES
1. Go for Greens! This smoothie is really good for adding greens. The sweet peaches and mangos are awesome with spinach or kale. Even my picky kids will drink them this way. (Especially if I call it a Shrek shake or Jedi Juice!)
2. Add Some Protein or Healthy Fats! This smoothie absolutely plays well with others, so I often play with the mix-ins. Some of my favorites are 1-2 Tbsp of chia seeds or a scoop of collagen protein. Collagen is flavorless and odorless and is a great easily digestible source of protein that we really like. If you're vegan or vegetarian, you'll want to stick with chia seeds (though I hear this is awesome).
3. Not a banana fan? No worries. Try subbing in additional peach or mango, or swap in something else–papaya, pineapple, passionfruit, or strawberries are all fantastic!
4. Get Creative. You can also get creative by adding a splash of coconut milk for some richness, or a squeeze of lime juice to brighten it up even more!

High protein acai bowl

Prep Time: 5 minutes
Total Time: 5 minutes
Serving: 1 serving

Ingredients
• 1 large frozen banana, chopped
• 1 cup frozen blueberries or mixed berries
• ½ cup plain greek yogurt, 0% or 2%
• 1 scoop vanilla or plain protein powder, whey or plant
• 1 ½ Tbsp acai powder
• ⅓ cup oat milk or almond milk
• Topping Options: granola, coconut flakes, bee pollen, chia seeds, sliced banana, strawberries, blueberries, cacao nibs, honey.

Instructions
• Add all ingredients to a high-speed blender.
• Blend until smooth and creamy. For a thinner acai smoothie bowl, add more milk. For a thicker one, add a bit more frozen banana or 1 – 3 ice cubes.
• Pour into a bowl and top with your choice of toppings. I love granola, banana slices, strawberry slices, coconut flakes, chia seeds, bee pollen, and a drizzle of honey. Enjoy!
Notes
1. Yogurt: I love plain 0% Greek yogurt, but any type should work. If vegan, use coconut yogurt or almond milk yogurt.
2. Frozen Banana: You can use a room-temperature banana. Simply add 2 – 4 ice cubes to make the smoothie bowl thick.
3. Protein Powder: I used whey protein, but you can use plant protein powder or collagen instead. Collagen has 30 grams of protein per serving.
4. Freezing: You can easily freeze acai bowls for meal prep. Simply prepare the smoothie bowl without toppings, add it to a freezer save container, and freeze for up to 6

months. When you are ready to enjoy your acai bowl, remove it from the freezer and let it thaw in the fridge for 30 minutes.

5. Make it Vegan: To make this acai bowl 100% vegan, substitute the Greek yogurt with almond milk yogurt, coconut yogurt, or your favorite dairy-free alternative. Also, make sure to use plant protein powder.

Berry Breakfast Smoothie Recipe

Ingredients
1. 1–2 bananas
2. 2 cups frozen berries
3. 3/4 cup coconut milk (or liquid of your choice)
4. 1/4 cup oats
5. 1/4 tsp. cinnamon
6. 1/2 tsp. vanilla

Instructions
1. Place everything in the blender.
2. Blend until smooth.
3. Enjoy!

Tropical Green Smoothie Recipe

Ingredients
1. 2 bananas
2. 2 cups kale
3. 1 cup frozen pineapple or mango
4. 3/4 cup coconut milk
5. 2 tbs chia seeds

Instructions
1. Place all of the smootie ingredients in the blender.
2. Blend until smooth.
3. Enjoy!

Protein Smoothie Bowl

Ingredients
• 10 ounces mixed berries
• ½ cup Greek yogurt unsweetened
• 1 scoop protein powder
• 1 tablespoon peanut butter
• ½ cup milk of choice

Instructions
• Add all your ingredients to the blender.
• Blend on high until smooth.
• Pour your blended smoothie into a bowl and top with your favorite add-ons (if desired).
• Serve and enjoy!

Recipe Notes
To make the thickest smoothie:
• Use a high powered blender.
• Use as many frozen ingredients as possible (add frozen banana).
• Use a little liquid as possible to blend
Ingredients:
1. Make-ahead smoothie bowl packs: To make a protein smoothie bowl freezer pack, freeze all the ingredients together in a bag or container (with an exception of the milk) and store in the freezer. When you are ready to enjoy,

add the freezer pack and milk to the blender, blend, and
enjoy!

STRAWBERRY BANANA SMOOTHIE RECIPE

PREP: 5 minutes
TOTAL: 5 minutes
SERVINGS: 2 servings

INGREDIENTS
• 2 cups fresh strawberries, halved
• 1 banana, quartered and frozen
• 1/2 cup Greek yogurt
• 1/2 cup milk

INSTRUCTIONS
• Add all ingredients to a high powered blender and blend
until smooth.

RECIPE TIPS
• Greek yogurt is nice and thick, but you could use regular
yogurt in this recipe as well.
• The Vitamix blender I use it the Vitamix Ascent 3500 -
and I love it!
• I also recommend these stainless steel straws and glass
straws instead of plastic straws.

PAPAYA SMOOTHIE

- prep time: 5 MINS
- total time: 5 MINUTES
- yield: 1
- category: SMOOTHIE
- method: BLENDER
- cuisine: AMERICAN
- diet: VEGAN

INGREDIENTS
- 1.5 cups cups peeled, chopped and frozen papaya (280 g)
- 1 medium frozen banana (100 g)
- 1/2 cup chopped carrot (85 g, grate if you don't have a high-speed blender)
- 1 small piece of fresh ginger, approx. 2 tsp if grated (optional)
- 1 scoop vegan vanilla protein powder (30 g)
- 1 cup unsweetened almond milk or another plant-based milk of choice (or more as needed)

INSTRUCTIONS
1. Add all ingredients to a high-speed blender and mix until smooth and creamy. Pour into a glass and enjoy!

NOTES
1. To freeze papaya, slice a papaya in half and scoop out the seeds. Peel and chop the papaya then freeze the chunks on a baking tray. Once frozen, store in the freezer in a freeze-safe bag or container.

Healthy Creamy Chocolate Avocado Smoothie

SERVES: 1
CUISINE: Vegan
CATEGORY: Smoothies
PREP TIME: 3 mins
COOK TIME: 1 mins
TOTAL TIME: 4 mins

INGREDIENTS:
• 8 ounces almond milk
• ½ cup crushed ice
• 1 ripe banana
• 3 dates, or 1 tablespoon honey
• ½ avocado (about ¼ cup)
• 2 tablespoons raw cacao
• 2 tablespoons almond butter
• 1½ teaspoon golden flaxseed

INSTRUCTIONS:
1. Blend for 30 seconds until smooth.

Orange Julius Smoothie

Prep Time: 5 minutes
Cook Time: 0 minutes
Total Time: 5 minutes
Servings: 2 servings
Course: Drink
Cuisine: American

Ingredients

- 1 cup ice cubes
- 1 medium frozen banana
- ½ cup plain greek yogurt
- ½ cup orange juice
- 2 teaspoons pure vanilla extract
- orange zest, from 1 orange
- 1 large orange, peeled and segmented
- 1 tablespoon ground flaxseed
- 1 teaspoon honey, maple syrup, or agave

Instructions
- Add ice, banana, yogurt, orange juice, vanilla, orange zest, oranges, ground flaxseed, and honey in a blender.
- Process until smooth, about 60 to 90 seconds.

Equipment
- Countertop Blender
- Decorative Paper Straws

Notes
1. Serving Size: 1 ¼ cup

KETO SMOOTHIE

PREP TIME: 5 MINUTES
TOTAL TIME: 5 MINUTES
SERVINGS: 2 PEOPLE

INGREDIENTS
- 1 cup cold water
- 1 cup baby spinach
- 1/2 cup cilantro

• 1 inch ginger - peeled
• 3/4 English cucumber - peeled
• 1/2-1 lemon - peeled
• 1 cup frozen avocado

INSTRUCTIONS
• Add all ingredients to a high speed blender and blend until smooth.
• Store in an air-tight container such as a mason jar in the fridge for up to 3 days.

Low carb blueberry smoothie

Ingredients
• 1⅓ cups canned, unsweetened coconut milk
• 3 oz. frozen blueberries or fresh blueberries
• 1 tbsp lemon juice
• ½ tsp vanilla extract

Instructions
1. Place all ingredients in a blender and mix until smooth.
2. Taste, and add more lemon juice if desired.

Carrot Smoothie

Ingredients
• 1 cup chopped carrots steamed and cooled if you do not have a high-power blender or to make extra smooth for kids
• 1/2 cup frozen sliced banana
• 1/2 cup plain Greek yogurt

- 1/2 cup unsweetened vanilla cashew milk unsweetened vanilla almond milk, or milk of your choice
- 1/4 cup frozen diced pineapple
- 2 tablespoons toasted walnuts
- 1 tablespoon flaked coconut optional
- 1/4 teaspoon cinnamon
- Pinch nutmeg
- shredded carrots, coconut, crushed walnuts for topping

Instructions
- Add all of the ingredients to your blender: carrots, banana, Greek yogurt, cashew milk, pineapple, walnuts, coconut (if using), cinnamon, and nutmeg.
- Blend until smooth. Enjoy immediately, topped with additional shredded carrots, coconut, and/or crushed walnuts as desired.

Notes
1. TO STORE: Smoothie is best enjoyed immediately upon blending. However, leftovers may be stored for up to 1 day in the fridge, if needed.

Peanut Butter Oatmeal Smoothie

- prep time: 5 MINUTES
- total time: 5 MINUTES
- yield: 2 SERVINGS
- category: BREAKFAST
- method: BLEND
- cuisine: AMERICAN
- diet: VEGAN

Ingredients
• 1/2 cup rolled oats or quick oats
• 2 frozen ripe bananas, peeled before freezing
• 2 tbsp peanut butter
• 1–2 tbsp maple syrup (optional but recommended)
• 1 tbsp ground flaxseed (optional)
• 1 tsp vanilla extract
• 1 tsp ground cinnamon
• 1/8 tsp salt
• 1 cup oat milk (or any milk)

Instructions
• Add all ingredients to a blender.
• Blend ingredients until smooth and creamy.
• Pour smoothie into glasses. Add an extra drizzle of peanut butter on top. Enjoy!

Notes
• I recommend sweetening the smoothie with maple syrup, but you can also add medjool dates, honey, agave nectar, etc.
• If you are gluten-free, double check the label on your oats to make sure they are certified gluten-free. Only use rolled oats or quick oats for this recipe. Do not use steel cut oats.
• Since they are optional, the nutrition information does not include maple syrup and ground flaxseed.

Blackberry and Yogurt Breakfast Smoothie

Ingredients
Makes 2 Servings
1. 1 banana

2. 2 cups (packed) spinach leaves
3. 1 cup frozen blackberries
4. 1 cup nonfat yogurt
5. 1/2 cup fresh orange juice
6. 1 teaspoon finely grated peeled ginger
7. 1 teaspoon honey or light agave syrup (nectar)

Preparation
1. Blend all ingredients in a blender until smooth. Divide
between glasses; serve immediately.

5-minute Kale and Spinach Smoothie

yield: 2 SERVINGS
prep time: 5 MINUTES
cook time: 0 MINUTES
cuisine: AMERICAN
course: BREAKFAST

INGREDIENTS
• 1 cup milk of choice, I used unsweetened almond milk
• ½ cup Greek yogurt
• 1 cup spinach, if using frozen, reduce to ½ cup
• 1 cup kale, stem removed, if using frozen, reduce to ½
cup
• 1 cup frozen mango
• 1 ripe banana
• 1 tablespoon peanut butter, optional

INSTRUCTIONS
• Add milk, yogurt, kale and spinach to the blender. Puree
until smooth and no chunks of greens remain. This step will

help ensure that your greens get entirely pureed so that you don't end up with a chunk of spinach or kale in a gulp of smoothie.
• Add mango, banana, and peanut butter to the blender. Blend again. Check for desired consistency and add water or some more ice and reblend if needed.
• Pour into two glasses, and enjoy right away.

Blueberry Spinach Smoothie (Quick & Easy!)

Course: Breakfast, Smoothie, SnackCuisine: AmericanKeyword: blueberry spinach smoothie
Prep Time: 5 minutes
Total Time: 5 minutes
Servings: 1
Calories: 334kcal

Equipment
• Blender

Ingredients
• ¾ cup blueberries fresh or frozen
• ¾ cup banana fresh or frozen
• 1 cup almond milk or any other milk
• 1-2 cups baby spinach
• 2 tablespoons lemon juice or the juice of 1 lemon
• 1-2 scoops vanilla protein powder or half a cup of Greek Yogurt

Instructions
• Add all of your ingredients to a blender

• Cover and blend until smooth. Sweeten to taste with honey if you like.

Notes

1. Optional Add-Ins: healthy fat boost: ½ ripe avocado, 1 tablespoon peanut butter/ almond butter fiber boost: 1 tablespoon chia seeds or ground flax seed sweeter: 1 tablespoon honey or maple syrup pinch of cinnamon. Nutrition information calculated using 2 cups of spinach, vanilla protein powder & almond milk and without any of the optional add-ins listed above. For a nut-free version, simply use any other milk (like traditional dairy milk or oat milk) in place of the almond milk.

2. For a vegan smoothie: This smoothie is naturally dairy free and gluten free, but be sure to use a plant based protein powder for a vegan version.

3. For a paleo smoothie: This smoothie is naturally dairy free and grain free, but be sure to use a paleo friendly protein powder for a paleo compliant version. For more ingredient swaps, modifications, tips & tricks (like how to make this into a smoothie bowl!) see the full blog post above.

Iron Rich Tropical Green Smoothie

PREP TIME: 5 minutes
COOK TIME: 0 minutes
COURSE: Breakfast, Drinks, Snack
CUISINE: American
SERVINGS: 1 large smoothie
CALORIES: 271 kcal

EQUIPMENT
• Blender

INGREDIENTS
• 2 cups baby spinach washed
• 2 cups kale washed, stems removed
• 1 mandarin orange peeled
• 1 lemon juiced
• 1 cup pineapple fresh or frozen
• ½ cup orange juice
• 8 ounces iced water

INSTRUCTIONS
• Put all ingredients into the blender in order listed above.2 cups baby spinach, 2 cups kale, 1 mandarin orange, 1 lemon, 1 cup pineapple, ½ cup orange juice, 8 ounces iced water
• Start blending on low speed. Increase speed to high once the spinach and kale start blending. Blend for 1 minute or until smooth.
• Enjoy!

NOTES

SUBSTITUTIONS
1. Iced Water – Feel free to use coconut water in place of ice water if desired.
2. Kale – You could use spinach only if that's all you have on hand.
3. Spinach – You could use all kale only
4. Pineapple – Mango would be delicious in place of pineapple
5. Lemon – Feel free to omit the lemon if desired

6. Orange Juice – Depending on how sweet you prefer your smoothie, you can omit or add more orange juice.

SMOOTHIE ADD-INS
• Hemp Seeds
• Protein Powders
• Banana
• Apple
• Coconut Water

Pineapple Green Smoothie

Ingredients
• ½ cup unsweetened almond milk
• ⅓ cup nonfat plain Greek yogurt
• 1 cup baby spinach
• 1 cup frozen banana slices (about 1 medium banana)
• ½ cup frozen pineapple chunks
• 1 tablespoon chia seeds
• 1-2 teaspoons pure maple syrup or honey (optional)

Directions
1. Add almond milk and yogurt to a blender, then add spinach, banana, pineapple, chia seeds and sweetener (if using); blend until smooth.

Mixed Berry Smoothie For Weight Loss

• Prep Time: 5m
• Total Time: 5m

• Serves: 1 serving
• Category: Full Body Cleanse Approved, Smoothies &
Juices, Raw, Vegan, Vegetarian, Gluten-Free

Ingredients
• 1 c homemade almond milk
• 1/4 c raspberries, frozen overnight
• 1/4 c blueberries, frozen overnight
• 5 strawberries, frozen overnight
• 1 banana, peeled and frozen overnight
• 1/4 tsp. cinnamon powder

Instructions
1. Add all of the ingredients to a blender and blend until
smooth.
2. Pour the smoothie into a large cup and enjoy.

The Weight Gain Smoothie Recipe for Kids

Course: Drinks
Cuisine: American
Prep Time: 10 minutes
Cook Time: 2 minutes
Total Time: 12 minutes
Servings: 1
Calories: 500 kcal

Ingredients
• 1/2 cup Whole Fat Coconut Milk
• 1 Semi-Ripe Banana
• 1/2 Ripe Avocado
• 1 tsp Vanilla Extract

Instructions
1. Add all main ingredients into a blender and mix on high until consistency is smooth.
2. Pour into a cup or bowl. Serve with a straw or spoon.

Recipe Notes
1. Smoothie can also be poured into popsicle molds and placed in the freezer.
2. Nutritional info is based on main ingredients. Chia seeds and nut butter will increase the fat, calories, and protein.

Optional Ingredients:
1. 1/4 tsp of cinnamon (can use more if your child likes this flavor)
2. 2-3 ice cubes (use if your child likes cold drinks)
3. 1/4 cup of berries (use for added nutrients)
4. 1 tbsp of nut butter (use for more fat and calories)
5. 1-3 tbsp of water or milk (use if smoothie is too thick)
6. 1 tbsp of chia seeds (use for nutrition and protein, but note it will make the smoothie thicker and possibly textured depending on your blender)
7. 1-3 tsp of cocoa powder (use to motivate your child if they like chocolate)

Easy Pre Workout Smoothie

Ingredients
- 1 ripe banana, peeled
- 1/2 cup frozen blueberries
- 1 tsp maple syrup
- 1 tsp cinnamon
- Juice from 1/2 lemon

• 2 scoops Naked Seed protein powder (or 1-2 scoops of protein powder of your choice, see notes)
• 1/2 cup unsweetened almond or oat milk

Instructions
1. Add all ingredients to a blender and blend until completely smooth.
2. Enjoy 30 minutes before working out for the best benefits (see notes).

Notes
• Choose from plant-based protein powders, whey protein, collagen, or egg white protein (see under recommended products and use the serving size as indicated on the container).
• This pre-workout smoothie is best for if you have a shorter amount of time to exercise or you are performing a fast high-intensity workout of shorter duration.
• If you are planning a longer duration workout (such as a 10km run, or another intense endurance activity of 1 hour or more, add 1/4 cup of whole grain rolled oats to your smoothie for slower digesting carbohydrates that provide longer-lasting energy)

Keto Smoothie Recipe with Avocado, Chia Seeds & Cacao

INGREDIENTS
• 1–1¼ cups full-fat coconut milk
• ½ frozen avocado
• 1 tablespoon nut butter of choice

• 1 tablespoon chia seeds, soaked in 3 tablespoons of water for 10 minutes
• 2 teaspoons cacao nibs, cacao powder or cocoa powder OR 1 scoop of chocolate protein powder made from bone broth
• 1 tablespoon coconut oil
• Ice (optional)
• For topping: cacao nibs and cinnamon
• ¼ cup water, if needed

INSTRUCTIONS
1. Add contents into a high-powered blender, blending until well-combined.
2. Top with cacao nibs and cinnamon.

CONCLUSION

The Volumetric Diet offers a practical, science-backed approach to weight management that focuses on consuming nutrient-dense, low-calorie foods that promote satiety and satisfaction. By prioritizing foods with high water and fiber content, this diet allows individuals to enjoy generous portions without the excess calories, making it easier to adhere to and sustain over the long term. The recipes and meal plans provided in this cookbook are designed to be both delicious and fulfilling, ensuring that you never feel deprived while working towards your health goals. By embracing the principles of volumetrics, you can cultivate healthier eating habits, improve your overall well-being, and maintain a balanced, enjoyable diet.

Remember, the key to success with the Volumetric Diet is mindful eating, variety, and consistency. Use the tools, tips, and recipes in this cookbook to guide your journey, and enjoy the path to a healthier, happier you.